Recover from Labyrinthitis and Vestibular Neuritis – Finally!

Marian Groome

Ambassador to Defeat Dizziness™

Vestibular Disorders Association (VEDA)

For more information about inner ear balance disorders, contact VEDA at:

E-mail: info@vestibular.org

Website: www.vestibular.org

PREFACE

If you have found this book, either you or someone you love are suffering with a debilitating inner ear illness. My decision to write this book was born from the frustration with the lack of knowledge, compassion and awareness from health care professionals, regarding the inner ear and people suffering from inner ear disorders. Any inner ear illness, however long it lasts, can be extremely frightening and isolating. I am in the unique position to pass my knowledge onto others, as not only am I also a sufferer, but I am a qualified Physiotherapy Assistant, hold a BSC (Hons) in Psychology and I am currently training in the field of Psychotherapy. This book will educate you on what is happening inside your body, the psychological and physical symptoms you are experiencing, how to avoid making your symptoms worse, and how to recover and maintain your health.

Contents

Chapter 1: My story 4

Chapter 2: Understanding the inner ear and the Vestibular System 16

Chapter 3: Most common types of vestibular disorders 19

Chapter 4: The main symptoms of Labyrinthitis and Vestibular Neuritis ..22

Chapter 5: Symptom triggers 28

Chapter 6: I can't get a diagnosis! 33

Chapter 7: Vestibular Rehabilitation Therapy 38

Chapter 8: Practical ways to cope with acute symptoms 43

Chapter 9: Coping with an invisible illness 49

Chapter 10: Coping with chronic illness 54

Chapter 11: Chronic fatigue 63

Chapter 12: Anxiety and panic attacks 69

Chapter 13: Maintaining vestibular illness – how to stay healthy 75

Chapter 1: My story

I will never forget the 18th of November 2010, the day my world changed forever. I was 27 years old. I was in a hotel with a friend having a spa night and I hadn't slept very well. For a few months, I had been on a diet that cut out wheat, dairy, sugar and caffeine all at once, and perhaps my immunity was low as a result of the change. I was under extreme pressure in my then job, working late hours with an unmanageable workload, and I was physically exhausted. At the same time, I had been experiencing some difficult personal issues, so I was also feeling very emotionally drained. I kept feeling slightly light-headed, but I assumed that it would pass and that I was just worn out. I had felt particularly faint in work one day and had to go home, but I put it down to a bad period that month.

In the week leading up to the 18th of November, I had felt very anxious and more exhausted than usual. I was a bit dizzy, felt faint again and began to get heart palpitations. When I sat at the breakfast table that morning in the spa, I started to feel extremely faint. I went outside for some air and my head felt very 'full'. I thought I was going to collapse. I went back to my room to lie down, but after a nap I didn't feel any better. I went home and for a few days I continued to feel lightheaded and tired. A couple of evenings later, I was in the kitchen talking to my mother when suddenly I felt the room spinning really wildly and I had to hold on to the side of the table. I tried to walk upstairs to my room but could barely manage. Lying in bed, I honestly thought I was dying. My whole body was shaking uncontrollably, my heart was racing, I was dizzy and disorientated and I felt I was sinking into the bed. The next day the doctor came to my house and she diagnosed me with labyrinthitis, a virus in the semi-circular canals of the inner ear. She said the symptoms could come on very suddenly and that I should be better in about two weeks.

The next month could only be described as a living HELL. I lay in bed feeling dizzy, and as though my head was stuffed with cotton wool. I was extremely fatigued and weak and was having panic attacks all day. If I stood up, my legs would shake so badly that I thought they would give way beneath me. Even if I merely sat up, I felt so nauseous and dizzy that it just wasn't worth it. My mother had to leave my breakfast and lunch on my bedroom floor before she went to work, because I was too dizzy and weak to go downstairs. My legs couldn't hold me even if I tried. If I needed to use the toilet, my mother had to walk with me, holding me up, one very slow step at a time. I had to cling on to the toilet bowl so I wouldn't fall off because the room was spinning so badly. Every day I would wake up to find that there was no improvement. I was convinced there was something else wrong with me and I kept looking up my symptoms on the internet. There was very little information available online, but anything I did find confirmed what I already knew I had – labyrinthitis, although the symptoms of MS and brain tumours are so similar that I was starting to believe I had those.

I kept telling my friends not to call to the house because I was afraid I would faint, become really dizzy or have a panic attack. I think one of the worst things about labyrinthitis is the anxiety and sense of panic. It's a very lonely illness, as you want to protect yourself from feeling dizzy, so isolating yourself seems the logical thing to do. It's hard to get back to normality when your head is cloudy and you feel disoriented and can't think straight. I ended up just wanting to be in bed all the time, as it was the place where I felt safest. This became detrimental to my psychological health. I was constantly anxious and would have a panic attack every time I knew somebody was coming to see me. The panic attacks made my vertigo worse. The two symptoms go hand in hand, with one exacerbating the other. I didn't want to tell anyone how bad I felt, as I wouldn't even admit to myself that I couldn't cope. I lost a lot of weight from the anxiety.

Very slowly, I became more mobile by forcing myself to move around a little bit each day. I pushed myself, thinking I would be ok, and I went back to work after about two months. However, I was utterly exhausted, still dizzy and having panic attacks, and I ended up getting worse. I decided to go to a party in a bar one night for a friend's 30th birthday, as I was so tired of missing out on social occasions and feeling isolated. The party was on the 3rd floor of the venue and I walked up and down long flights of stairs about six times, between bathroom breaks and going to the smoking area with my friends (even though I had given up smoking by this stage). On my last trip up the stairs, the room started violently spinning. I grabbed my friend to come downstairs with me and, sitting outside, I felt exactly like I had in the kitchen that night a few months before. She put me into a taxi because I felt so dizzy, nauseous, and anxious and I needed to have a sudden bowel movement. The taxi driver kept talking to me and I just kept thinking, 'please god, just leave me alone. I don't know what's happening to my body.'

The next day was back to hell again, it was as if I had just set myself back two months. I forced myself to go into work, but thought I was going to collapse a number of times on the way in. I had to stop and hold on to things so I didn't fall. I had honestly never felt anything like this in my whole life. The symptoms continued day after day, and after about six weeks in work I was so exhausted that I decided enough was enough. I took some more time off. At this stage, I was becoming terribly depressed. Before the party, I really had thought that I was starting to slowly recover, but now I was feeling worse every day. On top of this, I had visited two doctors who told me my symptoms were not caused by the virus as I was no longer feeling as dizzy. One doctor told me I had chronic fatigue, anxiety and mild depression, which had nothing to do with the labyrinthitis and would be cured if I went for a ten minute walk every day. Ten minutes?? I could barely get out of bed!! The other symptoms I was experiencing seemed to be taking over too, which made all the sensations in my head even more frightening. I was really starting to believe I had a more serious illness.

For the next few months, I was at home in bed on my own, day in, day out, and I was slowly losing my mind. I couldn't see a way out. My muscles were so weak from lying in bed all day, I felt as if I was withering away. I would book an appointment with a GP and receive the same reaction each time – a blank stare or an incorrect diagnosis. It was unbelievably frustrating and disheartening. I would look up labyrinthitis on the internet again, praying I would find some clue as to how to get better, but I found little or no information. The one or two sites I did find said my illness would clear up in two to six weeks. It seemed utterly hopeless. I remember lying in my bed saying to myself, 'I give up'. I didn't trust my own body any more, and I was frightened and sad. My life as I knew it was gone, and I felt trapped in a body that didn't work. I was so fatigued and weak that I remember one month, on my menstrual cycle, I genuinely wondered how my body could still be alive with so little energy. At the time, this thought was normal to me, as I had been so ill for so long. I also remember one day trying to change a pillowcase on my bed, but I was too feeble. Another time, I got so frustrated with feeling weak that I decided to water the flowers in the garden, as it was a beautiful day. Picking up the heavy watering can left me so fatigued that I had a sudden bowel movement and became extremely weak and anxious. I crawled back to bed shaking, disorientated and certain that I was dying – and I was ok with it. I just wanted this hell to be over. As I drifted off into what I had convinced myself was death, my only concern was that my mother would find me and she would be devastated. Other than that, I just didn't care anymore. I'd had enough. When I woke up an hour later and realised that I was still alive, I was genuinely surprised. When I thought back to those feelings about dying and not caring, I found it very traumatic. All this from a virus in my inner ear!

While I was going through all of this, my friends were incredibly supportive. All of them phoned and texted me to see how I was. They used to visit me even if I told them to stay away, and I was always glad that they did. One of them took me out for drives in his car and others just sat on my bed and talked to me even if I didn't really have the energy to talk back. Another friend had to feed me my lunch one day, as I was too exhausted to keep feeding myself. I got get well cards in the post all the time. I really felt so much love and support and I still feel blessed to this day that all of my friends were so amazing.

However, there were a small number of people who just didn't understand how sick I was and would say things like 'But you don't look sick'. One family member even said that they didn't believe I was sick. These comments were very hurtful, especially when I was at my lowest ebb and didn't have the emotional capacity to deal with people's ignorance. Coping with an invisible illness can be very draining, as you feel you're constantly re-affirming your illness by having to tell people that although you look fine, you are anything but. I often imagined, what if someone said to me, 'I have cancer', and my response was, 'but you don't look sick'!

By now, it was April and this had been going on for six months. I was crying all day, every day, as I felt I had no way out and that nobody could help me. I had tried a number of alternative therapies such as Kinesiology, but they had made no difference to my condition. I had attended seven different doctors by this point, had been tested for MS and for a brain tumour, but they had found nothing which meant I still had no diagnosis. I became very depressed. It was so hard going to sleep every night knowing the next day would bring no improvement. I couldn't believe I had been sick for so long. I felt so alone because nobody I knew had ever experienced this before. I felt all my friends were living their lives while I was stuck in my bed. I was missing out on so much.

Everybody reading this will have a different belief system or none. You may be atheist, you may belong to an organised religion as a Christian, Muslim, Jew, etc., or you may have your own sense of a higher being. I myself am not religious, but I do believe in a God. I had been praying and praying, asking God to help me, but I didn't get any relief. At that stage of my life, I was constantly reading 'Self Help' books. To be honest, I'd say I was brainwashed by them and their idea of the 'Law of Attraction' (that we attract good and bad experiences through the positive or negative thoughts we send out). Because of this, I truly believed that I had attracted this illness and wasn't getting better because I was a bad person and wasn't thinking positive thoughts. I felt totally abandoned by God, and my belief system at the time (which was made up of these books) was not working for me. I literally felt I was being broken down psychologically, physically and spiritually to my most vulnerable state. I would be rebuilt again much stronger than before, but I didn't know that then. For now, my whole world was crashing around me. I was trapped in a body that did not work properly and I felt I had absolutely no control over it. I practice Meditation every day and had done so before this illness. In my search for answers I spoke to my meditation teacher to ask her what the meaning of this illness might be, and why it could be happening to me. She told me a story about a saint who had also felt totally abandoned by God at one stage in his life, but that his experience was going to change things for the better. She also said that sometimes the journey of life is like being on train. Sometimes you'll go through dark tunnels, but you are still on the train, still on the journey. You will come through the tunnel and emerge into the light again. Another close friend told me a quote from Winston Churchill, 'If you're going through hell, just keep going'. That quote became like a mantra for me. I clung to this and my teachers' story because they were the only hope I had.

After about seven months, my miracle finally came. One evening, a good friend called to my house. We were in my sitting room when my sister-in-law called in and said she had the cure for me. I was so beaten and sceptical at this point that I actually said, 'I don't think it's going to work' before I even heard what she had to say. My sister-in-law is a yoga teacher, and after one of her classes she began talking to a lady about why she was attending. The lady mentioned that she had suffered with labyrinthitis that had lasted longer than the common two-week period. She gave my sister-in-law the number of a physiotherapist who specialised in Vestibular Rehabilitation Therapy and said that this would definitely help me to recover. When I phoned the next day, I didn't even know who or what I was ringing. I literally just said, 'I want book an appointment because I feel dizzy'. My first consultation was everything I had prayed for. The physiotherapist knew exactly what was wrong with me. She explained to me why I was feeling this way, what triggered my symptoms and most importantly that YES it was in fact my inner ear that was causing all of this and I would recover! I actually cried with relief when I left the clinic. She gave me a list of gentle head movements and balance exercises designed to get my vestibular muscles working again.

I began my exercises instantly but it took a couple of weeks to begin seeing a difference. However, I found over the next few months that I got worse before I got better. My vestibular system was getting to work again, which was amazing, but my fatigue levels meant I was completely bed-bound again and my eyes were extremely strained and sore. This meant I could not watch television, read books or be on my laptop for any longer than a few minutes. As a result, I was just lying in bed day after day, going insane from boredom and staring at the ceiling. It was torture. I was so frustrated that I couldn't just get up and go out. I found the anxiety and panic attacks got much worse too. I was afraid to do anything in case it made me feel worse. I had always been an extremely independent person, had never relied on anyone financially or emotionally. I had always liked to feel I was in control of my own life and that I could take care of myself. But when I was struck down with labyrinthitis, this mind-set was detrimental. I didn't tell anyone how depressed I was or how sick I felt. I kept putting my friends off from visiting because my hair was greasy, and I had no energy. I just wanted this vulnerable time to pass without anyone being any the wiser. But the more I pushed people away, the worse I felt psychologically, until one day I was so weak in mind and body that I realised I had no choice but to reach out to the people around me for help. It was the best decision I made. I knew from the way everyone reacted that I wasn't going through this alone. I didn't have to fake being ok. This was the best thing that had ever happened to me. I realised that we are not all invincible and that part of the human spirit is being vulnerable, whether we are male or female. There is nothing weak about it. It's a beautiful lesson I learned from this illness, that it's okay to ask for help. People love to feel they can help, especially when they really care for you.

I began tracking my progress in a diary every day. I would rate myself from 1 to 10 so I could look back on the bad days and see that I really was getting better. A really sweet friend made me a big sign for my wall that said, 'I AM GETTING BETTER', so I had a constant reminder that I was on the road to recovery whenever I was struggling. After about three months of performing VRT and slowly pacing myself to regain my stamina, I returned to work. I was still suffering from the depression, anxiety and panic, so I went to see a clinical psychologist who specialised in Cognitive Behavioural Therapy. She diagnosed me with post-traumatic stress, caused by the trauma of my situation. I attended sessions with her, actively learning how to change my thinking and really overcoming my depression. I am blessed and happy to say that for the most part, it worked.

I was terrified of my illness coming back and unfortunately, due to my lack of awareness about how to look after myself, it did come back about 7 months after I returned to work. I was 28 years old at this stage and loved to socialise with my friends. I was making up for lost time and drinking a lot on nights out, not getting enough sleep, not doing any VRT, and I was in the same stressful job. Eventually my body caved again. It wasn't as bad as the first time, but I was back to being bed-bound and extremely fatigued. I was referred to an Ear Nose and Throat (ENT) specialist by a new doctor. The consultant didn't tell me anything I hadn't known already, but he did refer me to an Audiologist, who performed a range of tests on my balance and vestibular system, such as position and eye movement tests. The Caloric Test was necessary but not pleasant – tubes are inserted into your ear canals to perform stimulus tests and assess nerve damage in the inner ear. It was here that I finally received my diagnosis. I have Bilateral Vestibular Hypofunction with 19% damage to my vestibular nerve, and my right side is weaker than my left. I had known that my illness was real anyway but here, finally, was my proof!

Psychologically, even though it sounds counter intuitive, I think the illness returning was the best thing that happened to me, because I learned not to fear it. I could trust that my symptoms were in fact my inner ear & not all in my head or a more severe illness. I had previously been hypersensitive to every single sensation in my body, but now these sensations were becoming familiar to me and I knew what to do when I felt really bad. I was sick for about six months more and needed to go through the whole process of rebuilding my strength again. However, this time the panic attacks were nearly non-existent because I had learnt how to change my thinking. I found I was more accepting of being sick because I trusted my Physiotherapist and the process of rehabilitation. I also used this time to really think about my life, in particular my stressful job. I had also been doing a degree in

Psychology part-time, so I made the decision to quit my job, get better, and finish my degree. It was the best decision I ever made. I had time to rest and give my all to my degree. During the second bout of illness, I began to really note what triggered my symptoms and I realised that I rarely felt unwell for no reason. It was usually when I pushed myself too far or forgot to perform my VRT that I got sick.

Over the next year or so I relapsed a few times, but it was never as bad again and usually lasted no more than a month or two. However, it was still disheartening and frustrating to feel I was taking 'one step forward and two back'. About two years ago, after a setback that lasted about a month, I decided to make changes to my lifestyle. I chose to give up alcohol, to sleep early every night, be strict on my diet, limit the amount of stress in my life (taking a lower-paid, less stressful job), be rigid about doing my VRT every single day and pace myself with exercise. So far, this has been my recipe for success. I almost always struggle with eye strain, and with fatigue and mild vertigo to some extent, but I can function in my life without letting these symptoms hold me back. Yes, I feel old before my time when I need to leave a pub before everyone else so I can get enough sleep, but it's a small price to pay for my health. Others don't have the worry of being sick for a week because they went for a jog and stayed out late on the same night. I try to ignore comments from anyone who doesn't understand, and also to realise that most people mean well. I know this illness is real so if people don't believe me just because 'I don't look sick', I really don't care. I am blessed with incredible support from friends and family, and I actually enjoy educating others about this illness. I am never afraid to talk about it, because who knows who I might help in the process?

This journey has been both a blessing and a curse – more of a blessing, though. I have taken so many positive things from being sick and learned to realise the valuable things in life, such as health, happiness and my relationships. I have chosen to change my career and to focus on helping the dizzy community. I have written this book, attained a Bachelor of Science Degree in Psychology, became a Physiotherapy Assistant (so I can perform VRT on other people) and am currently training in Psychotherapy. I always knew I would be led in a path for my career and left it to the hands of fate, but I never could have imagined the ups and downs I have been through to get where I am today. I still wouldn't change my experience and I fully believe this illness is not a life sentence. With VRT and some lifestyle changes, you can live a functioning life and be happy I wish you all the best in your recovery. Most importantly, never give up. You will get better.

With love,

Marian x

Chapter 2: Understanding the inner ear and the Vestibular System

The inner ear is located in the brain behind the cheekbones. It contains the sensory organs which the body needs for hearing and balance. It is comprised of three main sections:

1) **The Labyrinth** resembling three intertwined semi-circular canals which are filled with fluid and sensors and detect rotational movement of the head and aid balance. Each semicircle is at a different angle to the others and is responsible for recognising a particular head movement, for example, side to side, up and down and tilting to either side. In addition, each semicircle contains hair cells that are activated when the inner ear fluid moves. When our head moves, these hair cells send nerve impulses to the brain through the 'vestibulocochlear nerve' (also known as the acoustic nerve) telling the brain about the position of our head and body.

2) **The Cochlea (cock - lee - a)** which is a snail-shaped, bony structure filled with fluid. Hair cells inside the cochlea are the sensory receptors for hearing. The middle ear sends signals to the cochlea, which forces movement in the fluid that, in turn, stimulates the hair cells. Signals are detected from the fluid by the hair cells and are converted to nerve impulses. These impulses are sent via the auditory nerve to be processed by the auditory cortex in the brain. This is how we hear.

3) **The Vestibule** which is an egg-shaped cavity containing two sacks called the utricle and the saccule. The bottom of the labyrinth connects with the utricle which in turn connects with the saccule. The sensory cells located inside these sacks provide information about the position of the head when it is stationary. The utricle identifies horizontal changes in the body's position and the saccule detects vertical movements.

'The Vestibular System' refers to the inner ear, the eyes and the sensory receptors in the muscles, skin and joints, including, for example, the receptors in the soles of the feet. The overall function of the vestibular system is to process sensory information through the labyrinth, cochlea and vestibule, and to control balance and eye movements.

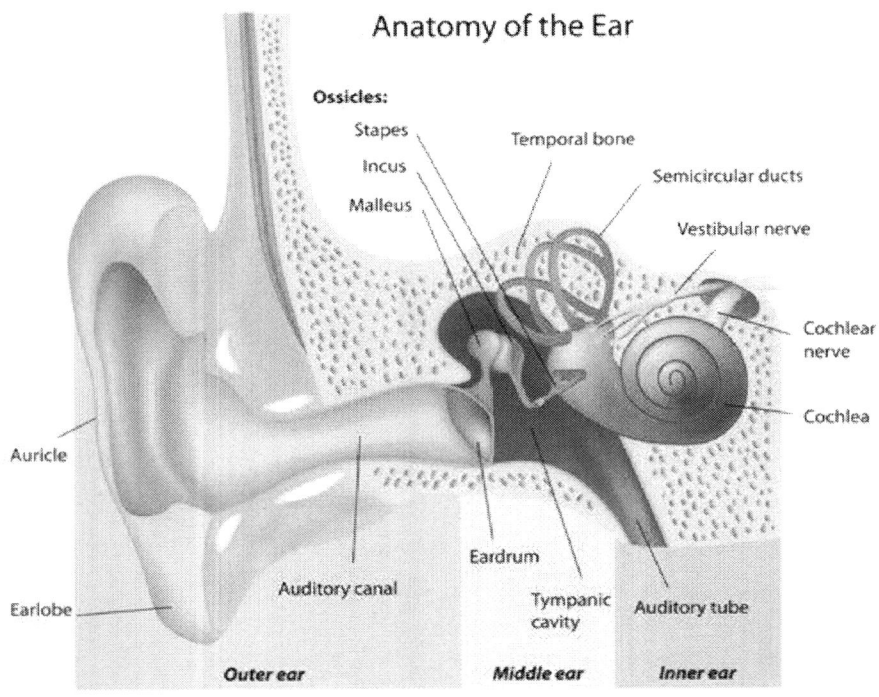

Figure 1: The ear

Chapter 3: Most common types of vestibular disorders

Labyrinthitis: A viral or occasionally bacterial infection causing inflammation of the labyrinth. This inflammation confuses the inner ear, causing it to send mixed messages to the brain about the position of the body, and creates feelings of dizziness and disequilibrium. Symptoms experienced include vertigo, tinnitus, and nausea and a person's balance can also be affected. There can be a number of causes such as a severe head cold or concussion. However, the most common cause is usually stress.

Vestibular Neuritis (VN): Affects the inner ear and causes the same symptoms as labyrinthitis. However, it involves inflammation of the vestibular nerve rather than the labyrinth.

Benign paroxysmal positional vertigo (BPPV): An inner ear disorder that causes attacks of vertigo based on the position of the body. BPPV is usually caused when crystals which line the inner ear canals become loose and send abnormal signals to the inner ear, leading it to believe that you are moving even when you are stationary. This causes the feeling of vertigo, particularly when lying down. BPPV can be caused from a trauma to the head (such as a fall), an inner ear infection, osteoporosis or diabetes.

Ménière's disease: A chronic and typically progressive illness which is caused by excess fluid in the inner canals. This fluid interferes with the inner ear's hearing and balance mechanisms, causing a range of symptoms, such as attacks of vertigo, hearing loss and tinnitus.

Unilateral/Bilateral Vestibular Hypofunction: The result of damage to the vestibular nerve endings – usually caused from the labyrinthitis/ VN virus, which obstructs the system functioning as it should. Unilateral means this damage happens on one side of the inner ear, bilateral means on both sides. The symptoms are the same as labyrinthitis. This can sometimes be referred to as 'Dandys Syndrome'.

Migraine-associated vertigo (MAV): Typically, this is migraine which is accompanied by vertigo. It can also be known as vestibular migraine.

Mal de Débarquement: Originally named for the sensation of movement after disembarking a boat, this is now sometimes used to describe a similar sensation caused by other forms of travel and other unusual motions, such as that felt after lying on a waterbed. Symptoms involve rocking, swaying, and disequilibrium which begin immediately after the event. Most people experience this sense of movement briefly, but for some it can last for a year or more.

Acoustic Neuroma/ Vestibular Schwannomas: A non-cancerous growth on the vestibulocochlear nerve that increases over time. Additionally, this growth can sometimes affect the facial nerves, causing numbness, weakness or a tingling sensation in the face.

Chapter 4: The main symptoms of Labyrinthitis and Vestibular Neuritis

Physical symptoms:

- Vertigo – a dizziness which feels like being drunk
- Spinning vertigo (dizziness like the room is spinning)
- Experience vertigo upon lying down
- A shaking feeling inside your head (similar to looking at footage of an earthquake)
- Tight chest
- Heart palpitations
- Shaking limbs
- Inability to stand due to shaking legs
- Feeling like you're falling over or losing balance completely
- Feeling like you're leaning/ being pulled to one side
- Unsteadiness
- Clumsiness
- Nausea and or vomiting
- Chronic and or debilitating fatigue
- Low stamina and weak
- Low immunity
- The ground looks like it's moving
- A floating sensation
- Light headed, faint, woozy
- Feeling like being drunk
- Sore, tired and strained eyes (which get worse when looking at the t.v. or computer)
- Pressure above/ in the eyes
- 'Flickering' or rolling eyes
- Unable to focus on moving objects
- Slightly blurred vision

- Stiff or tight neck muscles (this can increase the feeling of pressure and pain in the eyes)
- Heightened sensitivity to bright lights and sounds
- Headaches/ Migraines
- Head feels heavy or a very 'full' feeling
- A feeling of pressure in your head
- Motion intolerance
- Tinnitus
- Catarrh
- Blocked and popping ears
- Momentary deafness
- Hearing loss
- Pain in ears

Psychological Symptoms:

- Anxiety (Some sufferers report increased anxiety when eye symptoms are acute)
- Giddiness
- Panic attacks
- Depression/ Numb
- Frightening or disturbing thoughts/ dreams
- Vivid dreams
- Disturbed sleep
- Insomnia
- Trauma
- Mild confusion
- Feeling like being in a dream
- Disorientated

- Detached from reality
- De-realisation
- Feeling 'spaced out'
- 'Foggy' or 'cloudy' brain
- Unable to think clearly
- Slight memory loss

Common Emotions:

- Despair
- Depression
- Frustration
- Hopelessness
- Sad
- Helpless
- Fearful
- Abandoned
- Worried
- Emotionally drained
- Vulnerable
- Guilty
- Irritable
- Angry
- Agitated
- Overwhelmed

Common Thoughts:

- 'When will this end?'
- 'Will I ever get better?'

- 'Is my diagnosis of Labyrinthitis correct or do I actually have a Brain Tumour/ MS?' (as the symptoms are so similar)
- 'Why is this happening to me?'
- Worrying about the future - 'who will look after me if I don't get better?'
- 'Have I caused this illness?'
- 'I don't deserve this'
- 'Why has my faith failed me?'
- 'No one understands this/ what I am going through'
- 'No one believes that I am really sick'
- 'I can't cope anymore'
- 'I give up'
- Fearful of friends visiting you - 'what if I faint?'
- Unsure of what to expect with your body in the future
- If you're planning a family - 'how will I look after my new baby?'
- If you are experiencing a period when you're feeling well 'maybe I'm not actually sick?'

Common feelings and experiences:

- Loss of confidence due to loss of self-reliance
- Humiliated due to being newly dependent on others (maybe for the first time in your life)
- Embarrassed to ask others for help
- Feeling like a burden to others
- Nothing is spontaneous anymore
- Hypersensitivity to sensations in your head/ body
- Confused
- Feeling isolated and alone

- Feeling left out of social occasions or relationships with friends and family
- Not trusting/ understanding your body
- Extreme cabin fever
- Lack of trust in/ support from healthcare professionals
- Changes in relationships
- Unable to find any information about how you are feeling
- A feeling of one step forward and two back
- Feeling like this illness is always lurking in the background
- Feeling like a bad parent/ partner/ friend
- Constantly living with the uncertainty of when your symptoms will flare up
- Feeling lost
- Self-blame
- Withdrawing from your loved ones
- Actively avoiding places/ situations that make your symptoms worse
- Wanting to be alone more than usual

Chapter 5: Symptom triggers

Unfortunately, there are many situations which will aggravate and increase your symptoms. When the vestibular system is weak, it does not have the ability to process all the external information through the senses. For example, if you go to a supermarket and attempt to find something on a shelf, the combination of bright lights, rows of colourful products, patterns on the floor, loud background music and people talking, along with your own head moving up and down, is physically too much to process. Pushing yourself to be in an environment like this can result in a panic attack or severe anxiety, a flickering sensation in your eyes, or even the sudden need for a bowel movement. Such sensory overload can cause a setback in your recovery, as the vestibular system has been pushed way beyond its capacity.

It can sometimes feel as though these sensations are all in your imagination. However, you must remember that this is a very real illness which must be treated correctly. For example, if you had a bad flu but decided to push yourself before you were fully recovered, your symptoms would probably worsen. It is the same while you are recovering from this vestibular illness. Although you can be very anxious to return to your normal daily routine or duties, you must give yourself the time to rest and recover – even if it takes a few months. You need to acknowledge that your vestibular system is in recovery and the pace of your life needs to slow down immediately, to allow a complete recovery. The only alternative is to suffer with this illness indefinitely.

The following are symptom triggers (in no particular order of importance) that should be avoided where possible while you are in recovery:

Every day triggers:

- Looking at computer screens (especially scrolling up and down)
- Watching TV for long periods
- Spending long periods looking at a smart phone screen

- Standing for long periods/ Standing up too quickly
- Doing two or three things at the same time; for example, reading a book with the television on in the background on whilst having a conversation with somebody
- Conversing or laughing for long periods
- Hunger
- Tiredness
- Walking up long flights of stairs
- Riding an elevator
- Reading (especially small print such as a newspaper)
- Driving a car at night or while listening to the radio
- The movement of windscreen wipers on a car
- Being stationary for too long e.g. sitting down whilst travelling for long distances
- Reading whilst travelling i.e. on a bus/ in a car
- Patterned wallpaper, floor, curtains or clothes, or venetian blinds
- Colds or flu
- Rapid head movements
- Menstruation (obviously unavoidable)
- Watching a candle or fire flickering, or lights flashing or blinking
- Looking at light reflecting on glass
- Side effects of some medications such as sleeping pills
- Exposed ears on a windy day
- Getting water in your ears
- Washing your hair vigorously in the shower
- Drinking, smoking and recreational drug taking
- Lying down or rolling over in bed (mainly in BPPV sufferers)
- Rushing

Psychological triggers:

- Stress of any kind
- Constant worrying
- Anxiety

Exercise triggers:

- Walking at a fast pace
- Too much exercise, of any kind, at once
- Sexual intercourse
- Jogging/ Sprinting
- Gym equipment – but in particular the treadmill

Environment triggers:

- Crowds (for some of us, this can mean being around more than one or two people)
- Shops or shopping centres
- Anywhere with a lot of noise, loud music or people talking
- Anything with a lot of visual stimulus e.g. looking for something on a shop shelf
- Poorly lit rooms or being outside in the dark for long periods
- Cafes, restaurants or bars
- Busy public areas
- Fairgrounds
- Music concerts
- Stadiums
- Nightclubs
- The cinema

- The top seats in a theatre or arena looking down on the stage
- Anything that causes a vibrating sensation, for example, drilling, massage chairs
- Some bodies of water e.g. swimming pools or bath
- Watching the in and out motion of the tide or walking in and out of the ocean/ swimming pool
- Standing on an unsupported surface e.g. a decking
- Standing on a moving surface e.g. the inside of a train
- Walking on a travellator e.g. at the airport

When you are better you can slowly begin to introduce these activities into your weekly routine again. However, for now these should be avoided to prevent any further setbacks.

Chapter 6: I can't get a diagnosis!

One of the most frustrating elements of this illness is trying to get a proper diagnosis. You can absolutely still recover without a 'formal' diagnosis, but not having that diagnosis can be detrimental to your emotional well-being. You can begin to panic and think 'if the doctor doesn't know what's wrong with me, maybe it's something else?' When patients present to their GP with symptoms of an inner ear virus or bacterial infection, most will be treated with tablets for motion sickness such as 'Serc' or 'Stemetil'. These tablets aim to eliminate symptoms such as nausea or disequilibrium while the body heals itself. In some cases, this works, and the body heals within two weeks, with some patients even reporting that their symptoms had just disappeared overnight. For many sufferers, however, this does not happen. Sometimes inner ear illness can continue for up to six weeks or, if there is damage to any part of the vestibular system, for much longer.

The logical thing to do when we are still suffering the awful symptoms is to go back to our doctor. We trust that this medical professional will be able to cure us. We feel helpless and drained because we are not back to ourselves, and we are desperate to see an end to this misery. Some GP's will suggest some more time off work, while others might hazard a guess at another cause for our symptoms, such as chronic fatigue syndrome or depression. This leads to further hopelessness. Indeed, we may be suffering from chronic fatigue or depression, but these are symptoms or side effects of our vestibular illness not individual ailments.

At this stage, we can feel frustrated and alone. It is frightening to be sick for so long. The people around us are equally as puzzled that we are not getting better. We need to remember that doctors are 'general' practitioners with a certain amount of knowledge on many illnesses, but a lack of expertise on more unusual conditions. Often your GP may send you for an MRI scan in a hospital. This is where you are placed into a tunnel-shaped scanning machine which takes images of your brain. In this way, specialists can look for any damage, for tumours on the inner ear or an underlying illness such as MS (Multiple Sclerosis). In some cases, your GP may refer you to an Ears Nose Throat (ENT) Consultant / Otolaryngologist. The ENT consultant will attempt to find the type of dizziness you have. This requires performing some physical tests for example the 'Dix Hallpike' manoeuvre. This will show them if you are suffering with BPPV. This test involves, the client lying back on a bed and then being instructed to turn the head to the right or left by about 45 degrees. At this point the eyes will twitch or flicker, enabling the specialist to diagnose BPPV. A suggested diagnosis of Labyrinthitis, Ménière's disease, Migraine-Associated Vertigo or Vestibular Neuritis, will require an outline of your illness history and symptoms. Sometimes the ENT will refer you to a further specialist called an Audiologist, a specialist concerned with the diagnosis, treatment and management of hearing loss, tinnitus, and balance disorders. <u>Attending the Audiologist is how we receive our diagnosis.</u> So even if it's not suggested by the ENT, you can ask to be referred. Alternatively, you can skip the GP and ENT and book an appointment directly yourself. The Audiologist will perform a range of assessments to diagnose any damage to the inner ear which is causing prolonged symptoms. This involves hearing and balance testing and a 'Caloric test'. The Caloric test specifically examines the vestibular system and reveals any nerve damage in the inner ear. The test involves the consultant inserting tubes into your ear canals which blow hot and cold air or water into the inner ear, whilst monitoring any effects of the stimulation. The test will also diagnose whether the issue is on one side (unilateral) or both sides (bilateral).

Attending an Audiology clinic and receiving a balance assessment is the only way to receive an exact diagnosis. You don't require a doctor or ENT referral letter for an audiology clinic in Ireland, and in my experience these assessments cost in the region of 300 euro. If you can afford it, I would recommend paying for these tests as they will be able to identify what is causing the prolonged symptoms and will give you much needed peace of mind. In the back of this book there is a list of audiology clinics which perform balance assessments in Ireland.

On the basis of your results, it might be recommended that you receive Vestibular Rehabilitation Therapy (VRT). However, this is the most vital part of your recovery and the only way in which you will get better, so whether or not it is recommended for you, it is essential that you receive VRT from a specialised physiotherapist. Sometimes it's easy to think, 'if the doctor didn't recommend this, it's not for me'. The truth is, many doctors are not even aware that VRT exists!

When we start VRT, it is invaluable to have the results of our balance test from the Audiologist, so the Physiotherapist can design the correct programme to ensure our recovery. For example, the results of my own tests were 19% bilateral damage to my vestibular nerves, resulting in what's called Bilateral Vestibular Hypofunction. This means that I am functioning on 81% of my vestibular system on both sides of my brain. Based on this diagnosis, my physiotherapist was able to give me exercises targeting the weakest areas of my vestibular system. Please note that you can receive VRT and make a full recovery without attending an audiologist for these tests. They are not essential for recovery. However, for your own peace of mind, I highly recommend following this path to a diagnosis. On bad days, it's very easy to convince yourself that you're not suffering from an inner ear illness but from a brain tumour or MS.

So - the steps we must take to get a **diagnosis** are as follows:

General Practitioner (GP) who can refer you to an ENT (Ear Nose Throat) Specialist/ Otolaryngologist who can refer you to an Audiologist. Alternatively, you can contact an Audiologist directly to make an appointment. The benefit of attending a GP or ENT first is that they can send the Audiologist your previous test results or your illness history. However, they do not require this information to perform your inner ear or balance examinations.

What we must do to ensure **recovery** is:

Vestibular Rehabilitation Therapy exercises practiced daily at home, after an assessment with a specialised Physiotherapist.

Chapter 7: Vestibular Rehabilitation Therapy

Vestibular Rehabilitation Therapy may sound ominous, but it is simply a set of gentle exercises administered by a specialised Physiotherapist to strengthen the vestibular system. It is the equivalent of doing exercises to strengthen a muscle in your arm, for example, after it has been damaged. These VRT exercises are designed to increase function in all aspects of the vestibular system. The aim is to get us back to performing activities in our lives without dizziness or fatigue. When you first visit the Physiotherapist, they will perform an individual assessment to evaluate the severity of your symptoms. Based on this assessment, they will prescribe a set of exercises. They may also suggest temporary lifestyle changes, such as extra rest, until the vestibular system becomes stronger. Some people may require only a handful of sessions and others may need treatment over a few months. The therapist makes individual recommendations based on your response to therapy. The exercises they prescribe are a form of self-treatment and will be performed at home by you. The Physiotherapist will make sure you fully understand what you need to do before you leave their practice. Exercises are normally done once or twice a day. The Physiotherapist will understand exactly how you are feeling and can be an invaluable source of support while you are going through this illness. Do not be alarmed if your symptoms increase temporarily at the beginning of treatment, not everyone experiences this, however if you do, this is normal.

Here are some examples of the gentle exercises the Physiotherapist might prescribe. If you do not have access to a specialist Physiotherapist you can try these exercises at home until you can get an individual treatment:

- Balance strengthening exercises: stand on one leg with eyes open for 30 seconds, then repeat on the other leg for 30 seconds (twice daily). When this becomes easy, say after a week, perform this exercise standing on two pillows to increase the challenge.

- Gaze stability exercises (strengthening the eyes):
- Follow your finger with your eyes from left to right and back to left (repeat 30 times, once daily).
- Draw an 'A' on a piece of paper or cut out 'figure 2', from the end of this chapter, and stick it to a wall without a busy background, for example a white wall. Focusing your eyes gently on the 'A', turn your head from left to right and back to left (this being one turn). The aim is NOT to feel dizzy so perform this exercise very slowly (Do this for 30 seconds, 5 - 10 times daily). Perform these exercises particularly if you experience eye pain or sensations in your eyes
- Head movement exercises: Sitting down in an upright position, slowly move your head from left to right and back to left. Again, the aim is NOT to feel dizzy or any sensation when moving your head. If you feel dizzy slow the speed down until you feel nothing. (repeat five times, once daily)
- Walking: Slowly walk 5-6 paces, while turning your head from left to right and back to left at the same time. (Repeat 5 times, once daily)
- Turning: stand in one spot and slowly turn 360 degrees three times in each direction without increasing dizziness (once daily). Perform this exercise particularly if you have been feeling the sensation like you are leaning to one side

I must stress once again the vital importance of beginning VRT if you are experiencing chronic dizziness for an extended period after your Labyrinthitis or Vestibular Neuritis diagnosis. To target your specific area of weakness, you must receive an individual assessment from a specialised physiotherapist. Once you receive your individual set of VRT exercises, you need to perform them daily without fail. Performing them sporadically every now and then will not get you better. Think of it like this: if you had a bacterial illness and were prescribed an antibiotic daily for 7 days, you know that taking the medication on Monday, Thursday, and maybe Saturday would not get rid of your illness. Doing VRT is exactly the same. So, whether you have tried VRT in a half-hearted way before without results, or have never tried it at all, start as you mean to go on this time. Follow the guidance of your Physiotherapist/ this book to the letter. Trust that it will work. There is no other way to recover.

Not every Physiotherapist performs VRT because it is a specialised technique. To find your nearest Physiotherapist who specialises in VRT you can do the following:

- Use google search engine
- Contact any Audiology clinic or ENT specialist and ask them who they use or recommend
- Contact the Physiotherapy department of your nearest hospital ask them who they use or recommend
- Check the list of clinics in Ireland who perform VRT at the back of this book

For patients suffering with BPPV, the specialised Physiotherapist can also perform the Canalith Repositioning Procedure (also called the Epley manoeuvre) to reposition the crystals in the inner ear. This procedure usually involves the client sitting on the edge of a bed, then lying down on one side until the vertigo ends. The client then returns to the sitting position for a fixed interval and then lies down on the opposite side. These exercises are repeated in multiple sets throughout each day until the symptoms have ceased for a few days. For sufferers of Ménière's Disease, VRT can be very helpful between attacks to compensate for balance difficulties and can also be very effective in the later stages of the disease.

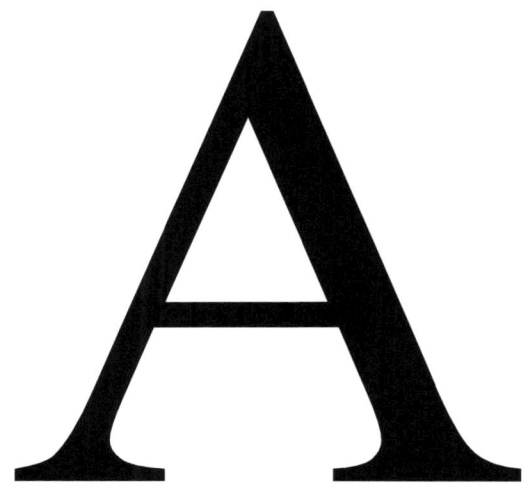

Figure 2: 'A' for part 2 of the Gaze Stability Exercise

Chapter 8: Practical ways to cope with acute symptoms

While you are recovering from Labyrinthitis, normal, daily tasks like visiting the supermarket or cooking may need to be modified or skipped altogether. Here is a list of practical ways to cope both physically and psychologically with acute symptoms:

1. Pace yourself, pace yourself, pace yourself!
2. Always know your limits when one or more friends call around. Talking or listening for too long can make you feel worse, even if it is only with one person. Definitely allow your friends and family to visit, but suggest that your time limit is, for example, one hour. They will understand.
3. As highlighted in chapter 7, if your eyes are very painful and sore try to refrain from watching TV, spending time on a computer or smart phone or reading, as these will increase your symptoms. A good way to relieve boredom is to listen to audiobooks or try audio of stand-up comedy to lighten your mood. If you must watch TV or use your smartphone for a short period, wear sunglasses to lessen the impact.
4. If scrolling on a computer is hurting your eyes, close your eyes as you scroll
5. While you are avoiding supermarkets, where possible, ask a caring friend or family member to order your groceries online to be delivered to your door. If you must go to the supermarket, it will help to wear dark sunglasses and to look at the floor as much as possible. Try to picture the layout of the shop in your mind when you make your list, so you get around the shop in the most logical order and make the trip as quick as possible.
6. If you celebrate Christmas, and are sick around the festive season, do your shopping online and get it delivered to your door. This might take some of the sparkle out of shopping for your loved ones, but the packed shops, bright lights and loud noise will be sure to set you back.

7. Where possible, try to avoid restaurants, bars and cafes. If you find yourself unable to avoid a special occasion or event, sit with your back to the surroundings – take a seat in the corner, facing the wall, so you will not be disturbed by the visual stimulus. Wear your sunglasses in this situation also and stay only for a short period of time.
8. Take time off work where possible. If you cannot take time off work during this period, ensure you take regular bathroom breaks during the day and sit for a few minutes in the cubicle with your eyes closed to rest the vestibular system. Make sure you rest during the day. Go somewhere quiet at lunchtime, even just to your car for example, and lie down with your eyes closed.
9. If you are sitting at a computer all day leading to sensations in your eyes, do the Gaze Stability Exercise (as mentioned in chapter 5) at least once, and massage the muscles at the base of your skull to help ease your eye strain.
10. There is a large body of evidence to suggest that the muscles in your neck can relieve eye pain and eye pressure. A deep tissue massage on your neck and shoulder muscles can help alleviate the pain and stiffness, and you can perform the massage on yourself. Covering your hands in oil and rubbing the muscles at the sides of your neck and at the base of your skull, can be very beneficial and can support relaxation as shown in figure 3, 4 & 5.

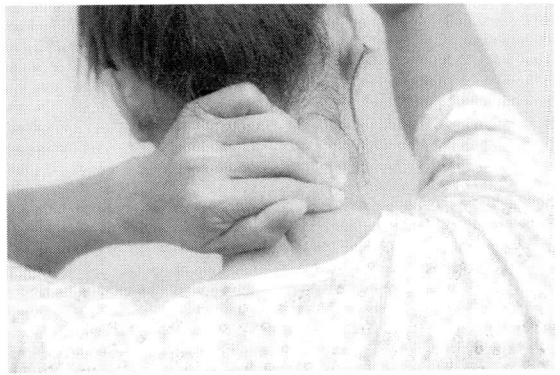

Figure: 3

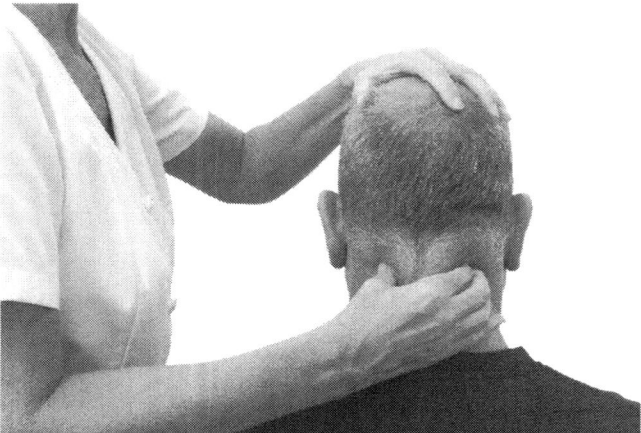

Figure: 4

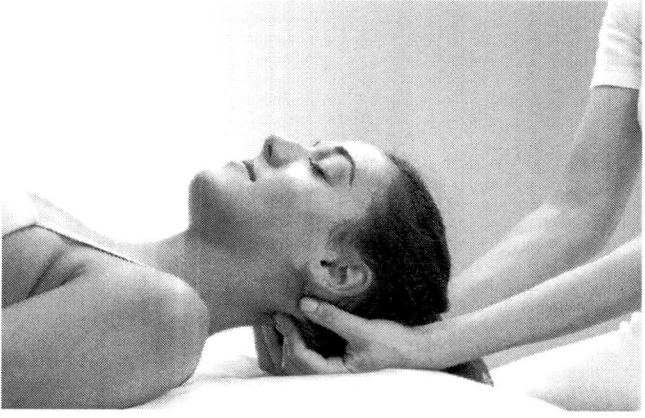

Figure: 5

11. Avoid places with poor lighting, as not being able to see the ground or surroundings will aggravate your system and could even cause you to lose your balance.
12. If you absolutely must go to a place with lots of noise; for example, a theatre, wearing earplugs can help to minimise the effect.

13. If hunger is a trigger for you, always have food, such as a banana, in your bag or pocket.
14. Avoid alcohol at all costs. Alcohol soaks into the fluid in the inner ear, and this can cause people to lose their balance. If the inner ear is damaged in any way, alcohol will place even more pressure on it and will result in a setback in your recovery. It's tempting to have a glass of wine or a beer to relieve stress or on a social occasion, but I cannot stress highly enough the importance of abstaining while you are in recovery. When you are stronger, you may be able to re-introduce alcohol slowly.
15. If you can afford to, hire a cleaner for a couple of hours a week to take the pressure off doing the house work.
16. If you have a dog, ask a friend or neighbour to take him/her for a walk. Many companies and individuals offer walking services if you can afford to pay.
17. If you cannot shower, try to wash yourself with a cloth and change your underwear and pyjamas as often as you can. It's surprising how feeling clean and fresh can lift your spirits.
18. Try to rest in different rooms throughout the day, to help alleviate feelings of cabin fever. Even if you live in a small house or flat, rotating rooms on a daily basis will help alleviate the feeling that you are lying in bed all day, every day.
19. Do something every day, no matter how small, to lift your spirits. For example, give yourself a gentle foot massage, light a candle or some incense, or eat your favourite food.
20. It's definitely important to talk about how you are feeling with friends and family, but sometimes it helps to talk about other things too. Chatting about what's happening in your friends' lives will take your mind off your suffering. This will help to lift your mood and fight depression.

21. Slow everything down. The pace of your walk, the pace at which you do things like shower or cook dinner. Rushing and stressing will increase your symptoms so, even if it feels unnatural, you need to slow down.
22. Relax. This illness causes a lot of anxiety, panic and fatigue so, where possible, lie down in silence for 30 minutes every day to rest the vestibular system. Put your mobile phone on silent and shut out the world. Take some deep belly breaths and focus your attention on each of part of your body in turn, starting from the feet and relaxing each part as you go. You might be surprised how much tension you are carrying in some areas.
23. If you have a partner and are feeling too fatigued for intimacy, communicate your needs with them. It might be helpful to assure them that it's not personal, but that you just don't have the energy at the moment for sex.
24. For women around your menstrual cycle take extra rest and acknowledge that your symptoms will increase for a few days. It's easy to feel you're taking one step forward and two back but try and stay strong: your symptoms will die down again towards the end of your cycle.
25. Keeping a short diary of your progress each day will help you to track how far you've come, especially when you're having a bad day. Simply rating your symptoms from 1 to 10 every day can help you to see any patterns or identify symptom triggers.

Chapter 9: Coping with an invisible illness

Coping with an invisible illness can be even harder than dealing with, for example, a broken leg. When the illness or injury is visible, people tend to have more sympathy as they can actually see the obstacles you are trying to overcome. However, if a friend or loved one looks healthy but complains of feeling unwell, it can be confusing. A natural caring reaction for many people is to suggest ways to help their friend, to show they care. When you are unwell, however, it can often seem as though those who are trying to help are being insensitive and simply don't understand what you are going through. On top of your physical, emotional and psychological trauma, you might feel as though you need to grow a thick skin! Some of these comments may sound familiar:

- 'But you don't look sick'
- 'Maybe you're depressed'
- 'Is there nothing you can take for that?'
- 'Why don't you get some exercise?'
- 'My uncle suffers with vertigo but he's fine'
- 'Why don't you try getting back to normal?'

These comments can leave us feeling unsupported or like it is our 'fault' we are sick. It can feel like we cannot live up to what other people are expecting of us, making us feel a sense of worthlessness or even causing us to feel depressed. If we are in a person's company who we feel does not believe we are sick, we can feel embarrassed and play down our symptoms. Sometimes it's easier to pretend we are ok because we feel too vulnerable to stick up for ourselves. If you are a young sufferer it can be even more difficult as sometimes others cannot believe a young healthy person can be so sick. It is a generally held belief that when someone young is sick, they quickly get better. So, when this is not happening it can sometimes lead others to question the authenticity of what we are saying. Additionally, we are missing out on many social occasions which can leave us feeling even more isolated. If we can attend social occasions but need to leave early or refrain from drinking, others may not understand and can even make insensitive remarks. Cancelling events can be extra heart breaking as others may not understand what it has taken for us to try and see them. Usually we have spent the whole day resting and avoiding doing anything in preparation, but our symptoms have flared up anyway, or through over exertion we are now unable for anything. This can leave us feeling so sad, helpless and frustrated and if others are dismissive or think we are lying it can be devastating. Some friends may not understand the nature of our limitations and even drop out of our lives altogether. Also, if you are single but would like to be in a relationship, you can even begin to worry that 'if this illness lasts I will never find a romantic partner' or you can have thoughts like 'nobody will put up with my illness'.

Then, when we are getting healthier and beginning to recover, returning to our old routines can give us a great sense of achievement. However, sometimes naturally our loved ones can assume we are 'cured' and not understand that we are still suffering with symptoms. It can feel as though we are constantly talking about our illness as we explain to people why we're not able for many social outings, long walks or late nights. It can be emotionally draining to continually point out what we cannot do anymore. After all, we are still trying to come to terms with our new limitations ourselves. Sometimes it can feel as if others don't believe us or think we are exaggerating how we feel because we don't 'look' sick. We can even go so far as to think, 'maybe they are right, and this is all in my head'. These thoughts can lead us to pushing ourselves before we are ready, making our symptoms worse.

What I must emphasise is that the majority of people mean well, want to help us and want to understand, but they simply lack awareness as they have never experienced a chronic, invisible illness before. This is not surprising, sometimes we may be unable to fathom an issue they are dealing with in their lives as we haven't been through it ourselves. But in our present situation, we can take control by changing our attitude and giving those around us the knowledge they need to help us. Here are some ways in which we can communicate with others and change our own thinking to help our situation:

- Communicate our needs to others, for example, 'I can go to the wedding, but I don't want to overdo it, so I will leave after the meal'.
- Be assertive in our communication.
- Show loved ones, friends or colleagues the parts of this book that are relevant to you, to enable them to understand what you are going through
- Be firm in what we are saying and let go of being attached to the outcome. If another person doesn't believe us or thinks we are exaggerating, that is not our issue. We know that what we are saying is the truth and detaching from another person's reaction can save us from feeling hurt or upset.
- Let go of expectations. Expecting a person to react in a certain way can lead us to feel even more let down and upset when they don't behave how we need them to.
- Try not to take it personally - some people genuinely mean well but can just say the wrong thing.
- If a loved one has un-knowingly made an insensitive remark communicate with them, where possible, that you found their remark hurtful and explain why. This way it can be avoided in the future and they will understand your position better.
- Confide in a trusted friend or family member.
- Know that this is not all in your head. You are suffering with a real illness

- Seek a good therapist who deals with patients with chronic illness.
- Show loved ones, friends or colleagues websites such as www.curelabyrinthitis.com or www.vestibular.org.
- Seek a forum online such as the one at www.labyrinthitis.org.uk where sufferers can confide in and gain support from each other.

Practising these ways of thinking and behaving towards others frees OURSELVES from the pain of feeling misunderstood, hurt or annoyed. We gain more confidence in ourselves and our bodies and feel less reliant on others for approval. We cannot change how others perceive what we are going through. If they think we are exaggerating or lying, this is not our problem. We know that how we feel is very real. From our experience, we can grow in compassion for others in similar situations, and blossom into stronger and more loving people.

Chapter 10: Coping with chronic illness

If this is the first time you have experienced chronic or long term illness, thinking about the length of time you have been sick can be frightening. It can almost feel like a dream – is this really happening? Whenever you are feeling like this, remember you are not alone. There is help out there. Many other people are feeling or have felt exactly the way you do now, struggling with hopelessness. It's natural to feel this way – your body is sick and you don't have the tools to fix it. When doctors aren't helping you and no one has any answers, it can seem like a life sentence. However, lying in bed day after day, spending too much time alone and not knowing when you will get better can be detrimental to your psychological state.

People with a chronic illness not only have to deal with the illness itself but also need to cope with

- The effects of the illness on daily life, for example, worries about paying bills if your finances are affected by an inability to work
- Changes in relationships with people around us
- Changes in how we live our lives, for example, having to stop playing a sport we love
- The psychological effects of being unable in obtain the correct diagnosis or treatment from healthcare professionals
- Side effects of medications
- Lack of support
- Depression & anxiety

The psychology of chronic illness is similar to that of grief. Grief is a natural response to loss and is the emotional suffering you feel when something is taken away from you. What this means is that the emotions associated with being chronically unwell, no matter what the illness, are akin to those associated with death. Chronic illness is a kind of death, the death of your old life as you knew it. From an evolutionary perspective, we can see how damaging chronic illness could be. If we were cave men or women, it could have meant not being able to provide for ourselves and our offspring, thus threatening our life and theirs. We still have these instincts, and they contribute to our difficulties in coping. When you look at it from this perspective, you can see that you are not weak or a failure for cracking under the pressure, you are in fact human, and very normal. There are, of course, other reasons why we find it challenging, but I am highlighting this one to emphasise that this is a very real psychological process that you are experiencing, and it is not all in your head.

Elizabeth Kübler-Ross, a Swiss-American Psychiatrist, first identified the five stages of grief in 1969. These same five psychological stages also apply to chronic illness:

- Denial
- Anger
- Bargaining
- Depression
- Acceptance

When we experience the death of a loved one, we may not go through the five stages in this order. Chronic illness affects us in the same way. We may float back and forth between all five stages at different times. This is completely normal. Let's go through these stages one by one:

Stage 1 – Denial: When we have been healthy and suddenly acquire an illness, it can be extremely difficult to cope with the realisation of what has happened. We can be in denial of how sick we are, or the length of time we have been sick, as a defence mechanism to help us cope. It can feel easier to deny the illness, for example by not looking after ourselves, rather than face the reality that we are sick and don't know when we will get better. If we have people relying on us, like children or an elderly relative, it can feel necessary to deny how we are feeling. Or you might feel as though the image of yourself as a healthy, active person will change if you accept your circumstances. You might be someone who has never even had a cold before, and here you are suffering for months with something you cannot control. You might feel like a failure if you accept your situation. Denial can manifest as thoughts like, 'I'll just keep going and hopefully I'll feel ok', 'surely I'll feel better by next week', 'I don't have time to be sick' or 'this couldn't be happening to me, I don't get sick'. Denial is a natural part of grief and can sometimes be beneficial, for example, it may give us time to slowly adjust to the realisation that we are ill. However, when we are in denial for too long, we stop ourselves from taking control of our recovery.

Methods of coping:

This stage is all about feeling a loss of control over our lives and our bodies. We can react by continuing with parts of our life that we know will make our symptoms worse, in order to give us a sense of normality. For example, we can keep drinking alcohol or pushing ourselves beyond our limits physically. However, this behaviour won't change the reality of what we are facing and will ensure that we continue to suffer. There are a number of ways to cope at this stage:

1. Talk about your fears and how it feels to be unwell with a loved one or therapist.
2. Examine exactly what it is about accepting your reality that you are afraid of, for example, 'if I take time out to heal my family will fall apart because I do everything for them' or 'the office won't be able to function without me'. Maybe in your situation you are putting too much pressure on yourself, and taking time out for yourself will not be as disastrous as you might think.

3. Really think about the consequences of not taking time to heal yourself and what that means for your future. Could you handle this illness indefinitely?
4. Write down any irrational thoughts you have about this illness or your recovery, for example, 'nobody believes that I'm sick so it must be all in my head' or 'people will think I am a bad mother because I don't have the energy to play with my children, so I'll just keep pushing myself'. Examine whether these thoughts are based on factual evidence or as a result of anxiety or fear.

Try to look honestly within yourself at why you are in denial. I understand this may be difficult to do as facing our reality can be very frightening. It can feel as if we are breaking down mentally, physically and spiritually. However, always remember that this illness is not a life sentence. If you follow the steps in this book, you can get back to living a normal life. You don't have to feel like a victim. You can choose to take the reins in your recovery, learn as much as you can about your symptoms and change your thinking to a more positive & hopeful mind-set. Working through your shock, disbelief, fear and anxiety about how sick your body feels, is vital in moving you out of denial and into another stage of grief. Difficult as it is to swallow, this is your reality at the moment. You can choose to stay stuck or you can begin to make decisions that will help you to move forward.

Stage 2 – Anger: Sometimes we can feel angry for 'allowing' ourselves to become sick or for 'causing' our illness. You can even blame a person or situation for making you sick, 'it is my bosses fault I am this stressed'. Listening to people complain about having a cold and being ill for a few days can be unbearable – if only they knew what it was like to suffer! We can feel angry that our lives are on hold and we are missing out, that people don't understand, that other people are healthy and they don't appreciate their health, that 'I don't deserve this: why me?'.

Methods of coping:

This is an important stage of grief and often one that can actually help us the most. Anger is a natural human emotion and should not be ignored or stifled. It can give us the strength to get motivated with our Vestibular Rehabilitation Therapy, for example. We can think 'I'm not giving in to this illness' and we can get our fight back. It is important to feel your anger and allow yourself to be annoyed. Yes, this is an awful illness! No, you don't deserve this to happen to you! The more you allow yourself to feel your anger, the quicker it will dissipate, making room for hope again. The important thing here is not to take your anger out on those around you who are trying to help. A healthy way of releasing anger is by screaming into a pillow or punching the pillow (if you can) with as much strength as you can muster. You will be surprised how much relief you feel afterwards. Another very effective way of dealing with anger is by writing it all down: all of your feelings, your angry thoughts and your anger at people around you - everything! Use every curse word you can imagine. Get all those thoughts and feelings out of your body and onto paper. Talking to a therapist is also a great way to express your frustration and anger with someone who is non-judgmental and compassionate. You are completely justified in feeling anger and frustration. Dealing with these feelings in a healthy way will help your psychological state while you are ill.

Stage 3 – Bargaining: This usually involves desperately trying to find anybody or anything (health professionals, God, scouring the internet for miracle cures) to help speed up the recovery process and change our circumstances. We would do anything to get our lives back again. We have thoughts like 'I'll try anything to get better' or 'if I get better I'll be super healthy and eat salads everyday', in the hope of bargaining with fate. We are under a dark cloud of 'what if's' and 'if only's'.

Methods of coping:

In this stage of our grief, we can feel panicked and desperate. We are focused on seeking any way possible to stop this illness from taking over our lives, even though it already has. Much like how we cope in with the denial stage, we need to take back control of our illness, physically and psychologically, and get involved in our treatment, trusting that it will work. We don't need to bargain anymore because we know VRT is our path to recovery. You need to really accept this and be disciplined with your VRT to ensure a full recovery. Yes, perhaps some of us may never be 100% well again, but after being so ill, we will happily accept being even 90% better!

Stage 4 – Depression: This can sometimes be the worse phase, the time when we just give up. We feel numb and experiencing any emotions seems like a luxury. We've tried everything to heal our bodies but nothing is working. Even mild depression can severely reduce our motivation to do anything at all, even to get out of bed. We can become withdrawn and isolated because we have just had enough. We don't have the emotional strength to stay positive or fight this illness anymore. The emotional torture of this illness is just as bad as the physical symptoms and we are struggling. The things that were once important in our lives – our relationships and our careers – no longer hold the same value. All we can think about or talk about is getting better. Our relationships suffer, but we don't have the energy or mental capacity to fix them. Sometimes we don't even care, we just want to stay in bed.

Methods of coping:

Going to bed night after night, knowing that you won't feel better in the morning, can be extremely difficult to cope with. The hope we gained in the bargaining stage has dissipated and we are in a state of despair, sorrow and numbness. Our life as we knew it is gone and there's no end in sight. We feel unwell every day. Our confidence in our bodies and our ability to perform even small tasks is gone. The natural reaction to feeling dizzy and fatigued all day is to isolate yourself and stay in bed. However, this is making the depression worse. It really is a vicious circle. Sometimes it is easy for you or your family to overlook the symptoms of depression, because it is natural to be sad and to cry when you are sick. Yes, crying and feeling sad are healthy ways to deal with your situation, but when these are the ONLY thoughts and feelings you are having over a prolonged time, depression becomes an issue. Both the inner ear illness AND the depression need to be treated. The good news is that both are absolutely treatable and there are a number of approaches to deal specifically with your depression:

- Talk to your doctor about temporarily taking antidepressants.
- Seek a Cognitive Behavioural Therapist for ways to deal with your anxiety, panic attacks and depression.
- Talk to a psychotherapist/ or counsellor (a non-judgemental professional who is trained to listen to how you are feeling).
- Do not isolate yourself - reach out to family and friends and let them know you are struggling. Build a support network that you deserve. Yes, you need to rest but you can definitely make time, in short bursts, for the people in your life. This is vital, so even if it's the last thing you feel like doing, force yourself!
- Talk to other sufferers on online forums or seek a support group in your area.
- Do something every day that makes you feel good, no matter how small. For example, give yourself a foot massage, put some perfume on, listen to relaxing music or to a 'positive thinking' cd or take a bath (if your symptoms allow).
- Make sure to talk to at least one person every day to stay connected to the people in your life.

- I recommend keeping a diary of your progress so that when you are having a bad day, you can look back and see how far you've come. This will help you realise that even if progress is slow, you are on the path to recovery.

Stage 5 – Acceptance: This stage will happen naturally over time. When we can accept the circumstances of our condition, we can begin to find more effective ways of coping. We can adapt our lifestyles to manage our illness and feel more positive about our lives and our recovery. This usually takes time, as well as knowledge about our condition, and what triggers to avoid. We may never be the person we were before this, but we can find a new self, with more compassion and understanding for others and a new perspective on life. We can take lessons from this and grow into an even better person! You might feel that you have accepted everything and suddenly go back to the anger or depressed stage. This is completely normal. When you can accept that your illness is manageable and that the symptoms are treatable, you will feel a sense of peace within yourself. That is when you can really start listening to your body and behaving in ways that promote your health, for example by avoiding alcohol.

Please remember that suffering from anxiety, panic attacks or depression is part of this illness. Intrusive irrational thoughts can also be present, and they don't mean you are 'crazy' or losing your mind. You are ill, so be gentle on yourself and follow the steps in this book. You will get better.

Chapter 11: Chronic fatigue

Dealing with chronic fatigue can be one of the worst aspects of this illness. As discussed, in the initial acute stages, it can be hard even to get out of bed. Gently moving your arms and legs is vital to keep your blood pumping around your body, avoiding clots and keeping your muscles and organs strong. It can be a good idea to wear compression stockings in bed to ensure blood flow when you cannot move around properly. The following are low-level exercises which can be performed in a chair or lying in bed and are designed for sufferers of chronic illness which causes debilitating fatigue:

- Foot pumps: Sitting on a chair/ bed place your feet flat on the floor. Raise your toes backwards toward you and hold for about five seconds, keeping your heels on the floor. Next, point your toes onto the floor and hold for about five seconds.
- If you are lying down, flex your toes upwards towards the ceiling and then downwards towards the floor, repeating five to ten times, depending on your energy levels. Afterwards point your toes downwards towards the floor and hold for about five seconds.
- Ankle circles: Sitting at the side of the bed/ on a chair raise your right leg out in front of you, slightly off the floor. Trace a circle in the air with your toes clockwise and then anticlockwise five times. Repeat with the left leg and left foot. These can also be performed whilst lying down by raising your legs slightly towards the ceiling and tracing the circles in the air.
- Leg raises: Lie down and raise your left leg off the bed as high as your energy levels allow, making sure you feel no pain. Hold for 3-5 seconds then lower your leg back to the bed. Repeat with your right leg.
- Shoulder rolls: Sitting in an upright position, raise your shoulders and circle them forward five times and back five times.
- Wrist circles: Lying down, raise your two arms towards the ceiling in front of you at the same time. Trace a circle clockwise and then

anticlockwise, about five times, with each wrist First with the left and then with the right.

Space these exercises out throughout the day and do them as often as your energy levels allow

The World Health Organisation suggests that an active body is the only way to prevent disease. By an active body, they mean a body that gets even ten minutes of low-level exercise three times a day, for example, by walking at a slow pace or lightly cleaning the house. When we are in recovery our immunity is low, so performing these gentle exercises will help fight off any other infections that we may be subject to, such as colds or flu. Therefore, it is important not to be afraid of exercise. Sometimes if we are having a good day and feeling like we have lots of energy, deciding to go for a 30-minute walk can seem like a good idea. However, by the time we come back, we are so drained and weak that we wish we hadn't bothered. This might cause our symptoms to increase over the next few days, making us feel even worse, and we vow never to exercise again for fear of another setback. What we must realise is that it was not the exercise that made us feel bad, it was the over-exertion, doing more than we were able for. Remember, pacing ourselves, even when we are feeling great, is essential. In this way, we get the vital benefits that exercise brings without making ourselves worse. Here are a few examples of how to pace yourself with exercise and lifestyle:

- If you need to go to the shops, bank and post office, don't assume you will manage all three in one day. Go to one of them each day or every other day, depending on your energy levels.
- If you need to see friends, make sure to rest for about 30 mins before you go if you can, and place a time limit on the visit.
- If you are very fatigued and need to cook a meal, sit down while you chop/prepare the ingredients and lie down while they are cooking.

- When you feel you are ready to begin taking exercise, start with a 10-minute walk at a slow pace. Don't exercise again for a day or two to see how you feel. If your symptoms do not increase, increase the time to 11 minutes on your next walk. Then increase to 12 minutes on the following walk and so on, keeping the pace the same. Always listen to your body and, if the extra minute each time is too much, go back to your previous time for a few walks until you are feeling stronger to increase again. There is no rule book with this. When you have built up your walking time to about 20 minutes with no impact on your symptoms, begin to slowly increase the pace on each walk but do not increase the time, again being vigilant with how your body is feeling. Always take a day between walks, e.g. Monday, Wednesday, and Friday and never increase the time and pace in the same walk. This is how slowly you need to re-build your stamina. It can be extremely frustrating, but it will ensure that you avoid putting too much pressure on your body. On the plus side, it can be very uplifting when you feel your body continually getting stronger.
- Never do everything in one day. Don't try to cook a time-consuming meal, go to the shops and go for a walk all in the same day. This can only be done when you are stronger.
- Always make sure you feel strong enough to perform an activity. If you didn't sleep well or have a cold and planned to take a ten-minute walk, reschedule to the following day. Never do too much when you are tired, thinking you will be ok. You won't. The exertion will aggravate your symptoms and will most likely cause a setback.
- If your eyes are really strained, restrict TV to twenty minutes. Increase to 22 minutes the following day, and so on. As I emphasised previously, avoid TV totally when the pain is acute.

Psychologically, this 'in between' phase can be difficult, as we are feeling well enough to perform some activities but not others. We can feel very discouraged and frustrated, as we just want to be normal again and resume our old lives. The saying 'patience is a virtue' is very relevant at this stage in recovery. You must keep pacing yourself and doing your VRT, reminding yourself, hourly if necessary, that you ARE getting better and just need some more time.

As outlined, always remember to plan your activities. Anything you need to achieve at the beginning of the week should be paced out over the seven days. As I've said before, rushing and stressing will increase your symptoms and maybe even cause a setback. It can feel as though the spontaneity has gone from life but remember, this will get better. Yes, you may need to manage your chronic fatigue in the long term, but as you learn about your limits, this feels like less of a prison sentence. The fatigue will lesson more and more as you recover. Over time, others will understand what you are and are not able for and will become more aware of your limitations. The most important thing is not to give up altogether! You just need to put your life on pause as much as you can in order to get better. Your vestibular system needs time to rebuild itself and pushing your body beyond what it is capable of WILL hinder your recovery.

Another thing to note here is that there are two types of fatigue. Feeling tired from a hard day at work is normal. However, feeling constantly fatigued or weak with low stamina, tiring easily after gentle activities or experiencing fatigue which is never alleviated by sleep, is the kind of fatigue I am referring to here. The psychological effects of chronic fatigue can be traumatic. Minor activities you never thought twice about, such as cleaning the dishes, have now become giant obstacles that you need to overcome without making yourself worse. You need to consider everything you are planning to do in advance, and whether you will have the energy for it or not.

You see friends and family rushing about and wonder where they are getting their energy from. If you have children, feeling guilty has become part of your daily existence because you simply don't have the energy to play with them, or even to interact with them in some cases. If you are in a relationship, it can feel that your partner is almost doing you a favour by sticking around. You can't go on dates, have sex or be your normal self. Your mood is depressed, and it seems as though all you are talking about is how bad you feel. The change in lifestyle and your new limits on shared activities such as housework or child minding can cause tension. This can really take its toll, so it's important to communicate with your partner about your concerns and insecurities. Yes, they need to be patient and to take over your duties while you are sick but assure them that it is temporary. You will get better by following the guidelines in this book and you will ultimately resume normal life. You may not ever be 100% well again but, by managing this illness, you can lead a regular life and follow a routine once again and, most importantly, you can regain your happiness and independence.

Chapter 12: Anxiety and panic attacks

The majority of people suffering with a vestibular illness report experiencing anxiety and panic attacks. Those who have never suffered from any mental health issues can find themselves gripped with panic on a daily basis. Feeling anxious is an understandable reaction to being dizzy 24 hours a day. However, there is plenty of evidence to suggest that the anxiety is caused by very real changes in the biological function of your brain.

The amygdala gland is an almond-shaped gland located underneath the vestibular system in the brain, and is responsible in part for how we experience emotions, in particular our 'fight or flight' reaction. When we feel fear or when a situation presents itself that could threaten our survival, the amygdala gland is stimulated, releasing hormones that cause biological responses, for example, increased heart rate and blood flow to the muscles, rapid breathing, diarrhoea and dilated pupils. We also experience behavioural responses such as trying to escape the situation. The body is preparing itself to flee from a scenario that might threaten its survival. This is a wonderful evolutionary response to being in danger, as it can help to save our life. However, it does not serve us when our fear response is being triggered constantly due to a biological 'malfunction', in a situation that does not threaten our existence. When we have a vestibular illness, our amygdala gland is constantly receiving messages from our brain telling our bodies that we are in danger. Evidence for this has been found in a study conducted in 2003 by Nakagawa et al. which showed that stimulation of the vestibular system was found to directly affect the amygdala gland, causing anxiety and panic attacks. Therefore, it is not all in your head, you don't simply feel 'a bit anxious' due to being dizzy. There are very real changes happening in your brain which are causing you to be in 'fight or flight' mode, 24 hours a day.

Unfortunately, what this means for us is that we have another element to deal with in our recovery. All we want to do is to protect ourselves and anything that will trigger your symptoms. You feel so anxious that a small task such as cooking a meal is too much to cope with. Even moving from one room to another at home can trigger a panic attack because you are out of your safety zone – your bed, for example. Having friends and family call to your house can be overwhelming. Allowing people to see you at your most vulnerable is not easy, particularly as a change in your environment can trigger anxiety or a panic attack. You can feel terrified of fainting or feeling dizzy around other people. You know your symptoms will be triggered so your 'fight or flight' response is on high alert. Your body is preparing for danger, so the natural response is to keep people away. However, if you allow these thoughts to consume you, the result is a crippling fear: fear of leaving the house or other comfortable surroundings where you feel safe, fear of exercise, fear of taking trips, fear of any change in your environment, fear of fainting, fear of falling over, fear of people thinking you are crazy or fear of people seeing you sick. If the anxiety is so intense that it is taking over your life, I would recommend asking your GP for something to alleviate it. I am not normally an advocate of taking medication, but the aim is to get you functioning in life again. If taking a low-strength Xanax, for example, allows you to have a visit from friends or to go for a short walk, it might be advisable. The aim is not to take medication over the long term, but to remove the symptoms of anxiety and panic in the short term, allowing you get your confidence back and to resume the activities you have enjoyed in the past. Over time, you will see that when the anxiety is gone, you can participate in activities that you had been avoiding. You will gain confidence knowing it is not the situation making you feel anxious, but the feelings associated with it. This can sound strange to someone who has never taken medication before, but while your symptoms are acute, and because the anxiety can usually be crippling, it is unlikely at this stage in recovery, that mental techniques will bring you much solace.

As you begin to regain strength and the dizziness is subsiding, indicating that your vestibular system is getting stronger, it would certainly be beneficial to attend a Cognitive Behavioural Therapist. The form of therapy is goal-orientated, specifically designed to give you practical techniques to overcome anxiety and panic attacks. The premise is that our thoughts, and not external events or situations, cause our feelings. So, the situation can remain the same, but we have the power to change how we feel about it, thus changing the outcome. We can learn, for instance, how to change our thinking about a friend calling over, so that it no longer causes a panic attack. With a CBT therapist, you can learn how to observe the thoughts and feelings you experience when you have a panic attack or feel anxious in a situation. Then you can learn how to overcome these feelings, so when they happen again, you can take control over your mind and create a different outcome, i.e., no panic attack. This will hopefully allow you to stop taking any medication you took to gain confidence in the acute stage of the illness, and to move forward by taking control of your thoughts and feelings. I cannot recommend this therapy enough and there is plenty of evidence in the fields of psychology and psychotherapy to show how effective it can be.

If you are not in a position financially or otherwise to attend a CBT therapist, Dr. Claire Weekes in her book 'Self-help for your nerves' describes a four step method of overcoming the symptoms of anxiety and panic. This method is:

- Facing
- Accepting
- Floating
- Letting time pass

Let's briefly look at each one individually:

Facing: acknowledge the sensations in your body, do not try to 'make' them go away. For example, you have felt the beginning of a panic or anxiety attack through sensations such as churning in your stomach, breathlessness, heart palpitations, trembling, giddiness, excessive sweating or any other unpleasant sensation that you associate with panic or anxiety. Understand that although you are feeling these sensations and your body perceives that you are in danger - you are safe. These sensations cannot harm you or kill you. Our rational minds understand that if you feel a strong sensation in your little finger for example, you wouldn't need to feel an intense sense of fear. You would know that it was just a sensation and you are not going to die or be harmed by it. Although it doesn't feel this way, it is exactly the same with your anxiety/ panic symptoms.

Most of us can develop 'protective' behaviours that enable us to feel in control of our bodies, such as carrying a bottle of water and taking a sip when the anxiety is acute. However, these behaviours can trick our brains into thinking they help to overcome the panic attack or anxiety but in actual fact we are fuelling the fire. What we need to do is 'Accept'.

Accepting: Do not fight against the panic - simply let go. Feel the symptoms in your body by putting your attention on them, knowing that you cannot die or faint and that you are not in danger. It will seem impossible, and counter intuitive, but as soon as you feel those symptoms, that is your queue to relax instead of tensing up. To remain tense, and 'fight' the sensations, by performing some of our protective behaviours or by fleeing the situation you are in, will only increase the amount of adrenaline being secreted in your brain and exacerbate the symptoms. By relaxing, letting go and not buying into the panicked thoughts fuelled by the adrenalin, the episode will be over quicker and not cause as much trauma. This may some time to master, but keep doing it, because you will master it!

Floating: Again, this seems counterintuitive, but continue about your day while the symptoms are happening. Don't resist anything or behave any differently than you would if you felt perfectly relaxed. 'Float' through the symptoms knowing they cannot harm you. For example; you are washing the dishes and your stomach begins to churn in the all too familiar way. Instead of panicking and feeding the sensation, calmly focus your attention on your stomach. Accept that the churning is just a sensation, it cannot harm you, you are not going to faint or die and nothing bad is about to happen. Then simply continue washing the dishes until the feeling fades. It is that easy. Repeating this way of thinking will train your mind to not fear these sensations, and eventually you won't even notice when it happens.

Letting time pass: Like everything with recovery from this illness, you must let time pass. You may feel impatient, wishing you could just feel better right now. However, this will leave you feeling tense and anxious, which are the opposite of what you are aiming to achieve. If you have a setback don't worry – begin the steps again. Persevere with this because changing your thinking can allow you to overcome this part of the illness!

Chapter 13: Maintaining vestibular illness – how to stay healthy

Once we accept our illness, we can learn to look after ourselves and our bodies properly. Read through the list of symptom triggers in chapter 7 and pay attention to which ones are relevant to you. Once you know what makes your symptoms worse, you can actively avoid the triggers. We are all individual and will have different triggers, but an overall way of maintaining your health is as follows:

1. Plenty of sleep. Lack of sleep will increase your symptoms, particularly eye pain, fatigue and vertigo. Prolonged sleep deprivation could even cause a setback.
2. A healthy diet is crucial to keep you strong and help prevent other illnesses such as cold and flu, especially now as you have low immunity while your body copes with the inner ear damage. Plenty of vegetables and oily fish provide much-needed vitamins and omega 3 oils for the brain.
3. No alcohol – this is essential. Alcohol is absorbed into the fluids in the inner ear causing temporary balance problems and other symptoms. If your inner ear is already damaged, it will struggle even harder to function, thus increasing your symptoms. Drinking a lot of alcohol can revert you right back to day one of your illness and may mean you have to begin your rehabilitation all over again.
4. No smoking. We all know the detrimental effects of smoking on our health, but smoking can particularly aggravate your vestibular symptoms, especially vertigo. Why not use this experience to start really looking after your body and to quit smoking for good? There are a number of tools to help you, such as Allen Carr's book, 'Easy Way to Stop Smoking', or you could talk to your doctor.
5. No stress, if possible. Stress is a major symptom trigger. Rushing when you are late, worrying constantly, trying to manage a huge workload or cramming too many activities into your day will all affect your health.

You need to start managing the stress in your life to make sure your symptoms don't increase. If you have a manager at work, talk to them about temporarily decreasing your workload, if possible. Take rest breaks throughout the day in work. Take more time out for yourself. PACE YOURSELF.

6. Relaxation. This goes hand in hand with minimising stress. It can be helpful to take up daily meditation. I recommend Transcendental Meditation, as this technique is simple, effortless and easy to perform. There is also a large body of scientific evidence highlighting the positive benefits of Transcendental Meditation on physical and mental health.
7. Perform your VRT exercises regularly. Depending on the level of damage to your vestibular system, you may need to practice VRT in the long term. Even when you are feeling good, always comply with your Physiotherapist if they advise you to do your exercises daily. If you have recovered and your symptoms have disappeared, it can be easy to forget to perform your exercises. However, failure to keep them up can weaken the vestibular system, leaving you vulnerable to a setback.

This illness is not like a cold where you can continue to push yourself and the symptoms will usually still disappear. Doing nothing to get yourself better in the case of a vestibular illness will ensure that you will suffer with this condition indefinitely. You must take control of your illness and recovery.

If you have had a hectic few days, for example, and you feel a setback might be happening because your symptoms have increased, you need to 'down tools', focus on and listen to your body. The more you are in tune with your body, the quicker you will become at sensing when your symptoms are returning helping you to prevent a longer period of illness. This does not mean you should become hypersensitive or panicked about your symptoms, but that you should check in with yourself regularly and be honest about how you are feeling. Don't choose to ignore any increase in your symptoms. Instead:

- Physically slow down, even the pace of your walk.
- Be disciplined with your VRT and even increase the daily frequency of the exercises.
- Get extra rest and sleep straight away.
- If you can take some time off work, I would suggest doing so until you are feeling stronger.
- Do not rush e.g. if you are late.
- Don't pack too much into your day.
- If possible, postpone any social functions until you are feeling better.
- View this as a mini recovery period until your symptoms decrease again.

You will notice there is some repetition throughout the chapters. This is intentional on my part as I want to highlight the importance of some triggers and life style changes that must be avoided while you are in recovery. I wish you all the very best with your recovery. I urge you to take control of your illness and make recovery your priority. You will get your life back.

REFERENCES:

Nakagawa A, Uno A, Horii A, Kitahara T, Kawamoto M, Uno Y, Fukushima M, Nishiike S, Takeda N, Kubo T (2003) Fos induction in the amygdala by vestibular information during hypergravity stimulation. [Electronic version] PubMed, Oct 3;986(1-2):114-23.

Physiotherapists who perform VRT in Ireland:

Dublin

Sandycove Physiotherapy, Sports Injury and Vestibular Clinic

The Forum,

29-31 Glasthule Road,

Glasthule,

Co. Dublin

Telephone: 01 2140575

Website: www.sandycovephysio.com

The Blackrock Clinic

Blackrock,

Co. Dublin

Telephone: 01 2832222

Website: www.blackrock-clinic.ie

The Balance Centre

40 Lower Leeson St,

Dublin 2

Telephone: 01 6625977

Beaumont Physiotherapy Department

Beaumont Hospital,

Dublin 9

Telephone 01 809 2526

Sutton Cross Physiotherapy

1 Sutton Cross,

Dublin 13

Telephone: 01 806 3030

Email: info@suttoncrossphysio.ie

Website: www.suttoncrossphysio.ie

PHYSIOFUSION

16 Warner's Lane,

Ranelagh,

Dublin 6

Telephone: 01-607-7104

Email: info@physiofusion.ie

Website: www.physiofusion.ie

Royal Victoria Eye and Ear Hospital

Adelaide Road,

Dublin 2

Telephone: 01 6644600

Website: www.rveeh.ie

Meath

Ashbourne Physiotherapy Clinic

9 Ashbourne Town Centre,

Main Street,

Ashbourne,

Co. Meath

Telephone: 01 8352043

Website: www.ashbournephysio.ie

Cork

East Cork Physiotherapy & Acupuncture Clinic

No 9, Cork New Road,

Midleton,

Co. Cork

Telephone: 021 – 4633 455

The Physio Company (various nationwide locations)

Telephone: 1890 749746

Website: www.thephysiocompany.com

Bon Secours Hospital

College Road,

Cork

Telephone: 021 4542807

Website: www.thephysiocompany.com

Galway

The Physio Company

39 Prospect Hill,

Prospect Medical Centre,

Galway City

Telephone: 1890 749746

Website: www.thephysiocompany.com

Waterford

The Physio Company

Waterford Health Park,

Slievekeale Road,

Waterford City

Telephone: 1890 749746

Website: www.thephysiocompany.com

Audiology Clinics Ireland:

Beacon Audiology

Suite 36,

Beacon Hall,

Beacon Court,

Sandyford,

Dublin 18

Telephone: 01 293 7930

Website: www.beaconaudiology.com

The Audiology Clinic

73 Lower Leeson Street,

Dublin 2

Telephone: 083 312 6299

Email: appointment@audiologyclinic.ie

Website: www.audiologyclinic.ie

The Audiology Clinic

Vista Primary Care,

Ballymore Eustace Road,

Naas,

Co Kildare

Telephone: Tel: 083 312 6299

Email: appointment@audiologyclinic.ie

Website: www.audiologyclinic.ie

The Audiology Clinic

Mallow Primary Healthcare Centre,

Mallow,

Co Cork

Telephone: Tel: 083 312 6299

Email: appointment@audiologyclinic.ie

Website: www.mphc.ie

Printed in Poland
by Amazon Fulfillment
Poland Sp. z o.o., Wrocław